The Anytime

BLOOD SUGAR LOG

Track All Day Without Limits

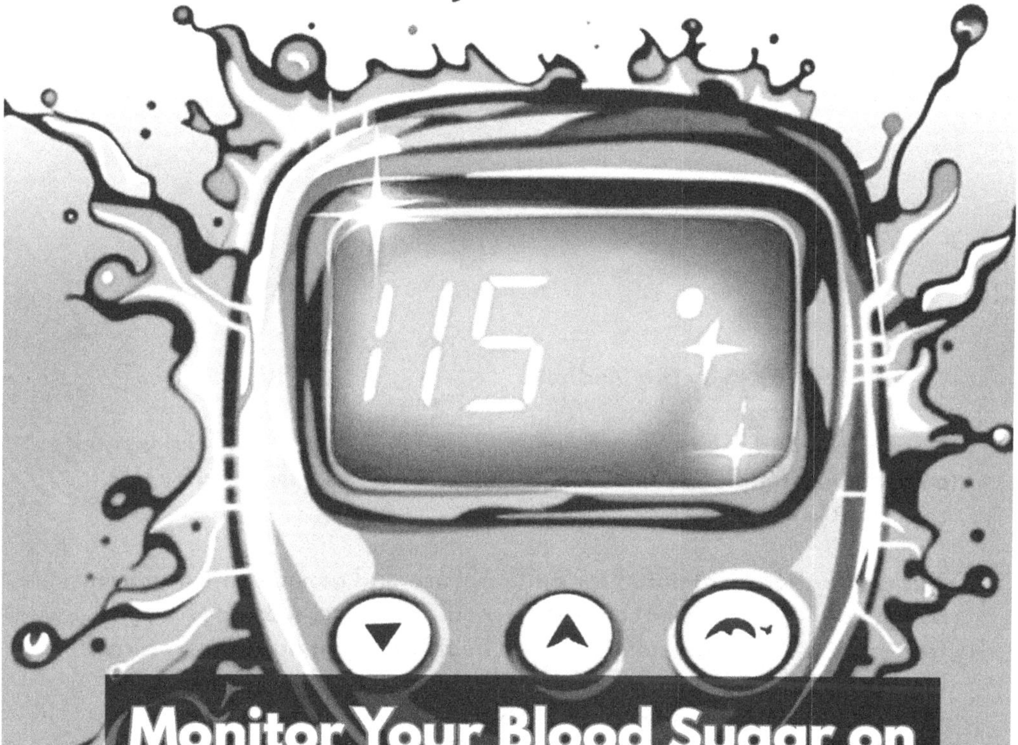

Monitor Your Blood Sugar on Your Schedule with Unlimited Tracking

DigiMedica

This publication is intended for personal use and general information purposes only. It does not constitute medical advice, diagnosis, or treatment. Always consult a licensed healthcare provider for medical concerns. The publisher and author disclaim any liability for actions taken based on the contents of this book.

PUBLISHED BY: ADALYNN JAMES PUBLISHING
Blue Ash, OH 45242
www.adalynnjames.com

ADALYNN JAMES

Glucose Monitoring Tips & Encouragement

Helpful Tips for Checking Your Blood Sugar:

- Wash your hands before testing to get an accurate result.
- Switch fingers often so one spot doesn't get sore.
- Check your levels as often as you need to. Before meals, after snacks, or anytime you don't feel right.
- Keep your supplies together in a small bag or pouch so you're always ready.
- If you see a number that doesn't make sense, wait a few minutes and try again.
- Note your emotions. Stress, illness, or even excitement can affect your blood sugar.

Tips for Tracking Food and Snacks:

- Eat some protein or fiber with carbs to help prevent blood sugar spikes.
- Pay attention to how you feel. Jittery, tired, dizzy—your mood and body signals matter too.
- Drink plenty of water. It helps your body manage sugar levels better.

Keep Going—You've Got This!

- Don't stress over one high or low reading. It's just information to help you learn.
- This logbook is for YOU. Use it to stay on track and take charge of your health.
- Focus on progress, not perfection. Small daily efforts add up.
- Be proud of yourself. You're doing something important for your body and your future.

"Small steps lead to big results. Keep moving forward."

— DigiMedical, by Adalynn James Publishing

⚠ When to Get Help ⚠

Sometimes, blood sugar levels can be dangerous. It's important to know when to call 911 or get medical help right away.

Call 911 or get help if:

- Your blood sugar is below 55 mg/dL and won't go up after eating or drinking something sugary.
- Your blood sugar is over 350 mg/dL and won't go down, even with insulin. (Your doctor may give you a different range of target numbers.)
- You pass out, faint or feel like you're about to faint.
- You feel confused and can't think clearly.
- You have a seizure (Your body shakes and you can't stop it.)
- You throw up more than once and can't keep food or drinks down.
- Feel very short of breath or have chest pain.

Important:

- If something feels wrong, don't wait. It's better to be safe and get help. Call 911 or go to the ER.

Notes about any reactions or questions to ask the doctor:

____

____

____

BLOOD SUGAR LOG

Month: ____________________ **WEEK OF:** ____________________

DATE	TIME	PRE-MEAL BLOOD SUGAR	INSULIN TAKEN?	BLOOD SUGAR 2 HRS LATER	INSULIN TAKEN?

BLOOD SUGAR LOG

Month: ______________________ **WEEK OF:** ______________________

DATE	TIME	PRE-MEAL BLOOD SUGAR	INSULIN TAKEN?	BLOOD SUGAR 2 HRS LATER	INSULIN TAKEN?

BLOOD SUGAR LOG

Month: ____________________ **WEEK OF:** ____________________

DATE	TIME	PRE-MEAL BLOOD SUGAR	INSULIN TAKEN?	BLOOD SUGAR 2 HRS LATER	INSULIN TAKEN?

BLOOD SUGAR LOG

Month: ______________________ **WEEK OF:** ______________________

DATE	TIME	PRE-MEAL BLOOD SUGAR	INSULIN TAKEN?	BLOOD SUGAR 2 HRS LATER	INSULIN TAKEN?

BLOOD SUGAR LOG

Month: ______________________ **WEEK OF:** ______________________

DATE	TIME	PRE-MEAL BLOOD SUGAR	INSULIN TAKEN?	BLOOD SUGAR 2 HRS LATER	INSULIN TAKEN?

BLOOD SUGAR LOG

Month: ______________________ **WEEK OF:** ____________________

DATE	TIME	PRE-MEAL BLOOD SUGAR	INSULIN TAKEN?	BLOOD SUGAR 2 HRS LATER	INSULIN TAKEN?

BLOOD SUGAR LOG

Month: ______________________ **WEEK OF:** ______________________

DATE	TIME	PRE-MEAL BLOOD SUGAR	INSULIN TAKEN?	BLOOD SUGAR 2 HRS LATER	INSULIN TAKEN?

BLOOD SUGAR LOG

Month: ______________________ **WEEK OF:** ________________

DATE	TIME	PRE-MEAL BLOOD SUGAR	INSULIN TAKEN?	BLOOD SUGAR 2 HRS LATER	INSULIN TAKEN?

BLOOD SUGAR LOG

Month: ____________________ **WEEK OF:** ____________________

DATE	TIME	PRE-MEAL BLOOD SUGAR	INSULIN TAKEN?	BLOOD SUGAR 2 HRS LATER	INSULIN TAKEN?

BLOOD SUGAR LOG

Month: ______________________ **WEEK OF:** ______________________

DATE	TIME	PRE-MEAL BLOOD SUGAR	INSULIN TAKEN?	BLOOD SUGAR 2 HRS LATER	INSULIN TAKEN?

BLOOD SUGAR LOG

Month: ______________________ **WEEK OF:** ______________________

DATE	TIME	PRE-MEAL BLOOD SUGAR	INSULIN TAKEN?	BLOOD SUGAR 2 HRS LATER	INSULIN TAKEN?

BLOOD SUGAR LOG

Month: ______________________ **WEEK OF:** ______________________

DATE	TIME	PRE-MEAL BLOOD SUGAR	INSULIN TAKEN?	BLOOD SUGAR 2 HRS LATER	INSULIN TAKEN?

BLOOD SUGAR LOG

Month: ____________________ **WEEK OF:** ____________________

DATE	TIME	PRE-MEAL BLOOD SUGAR	INSULIN TAKEN?	BLOOD SUGAR 2 HRS LATER	INSULIN TAKEN?

BLOOD SUGAR LOG

Month: ____________________ WEEK OF: ____________________

DATE	TIME	PRE-MEAL BLOOD SUGAR	INSULIN TAKEN?	BLOOD SUGAR 2 HRS LATER	INSULIN TAKEN?

BLOOD SUGAR LOG

Month: ____________________ **WEEK OF:** ____________________

DATE	TIME	PRE-MEAL BLOOD SUGAR	INSULIN TAKEN?	BLOOD SUGAR 2 HRS LATER	INSULIN TAKEN?

BLOOD SUGAR LOG

Month: ____________________ **WEEK OF:** ____________________

DATE	TIME	PRE-MEAL BLOOD SUGAR	INSULIN TAKEN?	BLOOD SUGAR 2 HRS LATER	INSULIN TAKEN?

BLOOD SUGAR LOG

Month: ____________________ **WEEK OF:** ____________________

DATE	TIME	PRE-MEAL BLOOD SUGAR	INSULIN TAKEN?	BLOOD SUGAR 2 HRS LATER	INSULIN TAKEN?

BLOOD SUGAR LOG

Month: ______________________ **WEEK OF:** ______________________

DATE	TIME	PRE-MEAL BLOOD SUGAR	INSULIN TAKEN?	BLOOD SUGAR 2 HRS LATER	INSULIN TAKEN?

BLOOD SUGAR LOG

Month: ____________________ **WEEK OF:** ____________________

DATE	TIME	PRE-MEAL BLOOD SUGAR	INSULIN TAKEN?	BLOOD SUGAR 2 HRS LATER	INSULIN TAKEN?

BLOOD SUGAR LOG

Month: ______________________ **WEEK OF:** ______________________

DATE	TIME	PRE-MEAL BLOOD SUGAR	INSULIN TAKEN?	BLOOD SUGAR 2 HRS LATER	INSULIN TAKEN?

BLOOD SUGAR LOG

Month: ______________________ **WEEK OF:** ______________________

DATE	TIME	PRE-MEAL BLOOD SUGAR	INSULIN TAKEN?	BLOOD SUGAR 2 HRS LATER	INSULIN TAKEN?

BLOOD SUGAR LOG

Month: ______________________ **WEEK OF:** ______________________

DATE	TIME	PRE-MEAL BLOOD SUGAR	INSULIN TAKEN?	BLOOD SUGAR 2 HRS LATER	INSULIN TAKEN?

BLOOD SUGAR LOG

Month: ______________________ **WEEK OF:** ______________________

DATE	TIME	PRE-MEAL BLOOD SUGAR	INSULIN TAKEN?	BLOOD SUGAR 2 HRS LATER	INSULIN TAKEN?

BLOOD SUGAR LOG

Month: ______________________ **WEEK OF:** ______________________

DATE	TIME	PRE-MEAL BLOOD SUGAR	INSULIN TAKEN?	BLOOD SUGAR 2 HRS LATER	INSULIN TAKEN?

BLOOD SUGAR LOG

Month: ______________________ **WEEK OF:** ______________________

DATE	TIME	PRE-MEAL BLOOD SUGAR	INSULIN TAKEN?	BLOOD SUGAR 2 HRS LATER	INSULIN TAKEN?

BLOOD SUGAR LOG

Month: ______________________ **WEEK OF:** ______________________

DATE	TIME	PRE-MEAL BLOOD SUGAR	INSULIN TAKEN?	BLOOD SUGAR 2 HRS LATER	INSULIN TAKEN?

BLOOD SUGAR LOG

Month: ____________________ **WEEK OF:** ____________________

DATE	TIME	PRE-MEAL BLOOD SUGAR	INSULIN TAKEN?	BLOOD SUGAR 2 HRS LATER	INSULIN TAKEN?

BLOOD SUGAR LOG

Month: ______________________________ **WEEK OF:** ______________________

DATE	TIME	PRE-MEAL BLOOD SUGAR	INSULIN TAKEN?	BLOOD SUGAR 2 HRS LATER	INSULIN TAKEN?

BLOOD SUGAR LOG

Month: ______________________ **WEEK OF:** ______________________

DATE	TIME	PRE-MEAL BLOOD SUGAR	INSULIN TAKEN?	BLOOD SUGAR 2 HRS LATER	INSULIN TAKEN?

BLOOD SUGAR LOG

Month: ______________________________ **WEEK OF:** ______________________

DATE	TIME	PRE-MEAL BLOOD SUGAR	INSULIN TAKEN?	BLOOD SUGAR 2 HRS LATER	INSULIN TAKEN?

BLOOD SUGAR LOG

Month: ____________________ **WEEK OF:** ____________________

DATE	TIME	PRE-MEAL BLOOD SUGAR	INSULIN TAKEN?	BLOOD SUGAR 2 HRS LATER	INSULIN TAKEN?

BLOOD SUGAR LOG

Month: ____________________ **WEEK OF:** ____________________

DATE	TIME	PRE-MEAL BLOOD SUGAR	INSULIN TAKEN?	BLOOD SUGAR 2 HRS LATER	INSULIN TAKEN?

BLOOD SUGAR LOG

Month: ______________________ **WEEK OF:** ______________________

DATE	TIME	PRE-MEAL BLOOD SUGAR	INSULIN TAKEN?	BLOOD SUGAR 2 HRS LATER	INSULIN TAKEN?

BLOOD SUGAR LOG

Month: ____________________ **WEEK OF:** ____________________

DATE	TIME	PRE-MEAL BLOOD SUGAR	INSULIN TAKEN?	BLOOD SUGAR 2 HRS LATER	INSULIN TAKEN?

BLOOD SUGAR LOG

Month: ______________________ **WEEK OF:** ______________________

DATE	TIME	PRE-MEAL BLOOD SUGAR	INSULIN TAKEN?	BLOOD SUGAR 2 HRS LATER	INSULIN TAKEN?

BLOOD SUGAR LOG

Month: ____________________ **WEEK OF:** ____________________

DATE	TIME	PRE-MEAL BLOOD SUGAR	INSULIN TAKEN?	BLOOD SUGAR 2 HRS LATER	INSULIN TAKEN?

BLOOD SUGAR LOG

Month: ______________________ **WEEK OF:** ______________________

DATE	TIME	PRE-MEAL BLOOD SUGAR	INSULIN TAKEN?	BLOOD SUGAR 2 HRS LATER	INSULIN TAKEN?

BLOOD SUGAR LOG

Month: ______________________ **WEEK OF:** ______________________

DATE	TIME	PRE-MEAL BLOOD SUGAR	INSULIN TAKEN?	BLOOD SUGAR 2 HRS LATER	INSULIN TAKEN?

BLOOD SUGAR LOG

Month: ____________________ **WEEK OF:** ____________________

DATE	TIME	PRE-MEAL BLOOD SUGAR	INSULIN TAKEN?	BLOOD SUGAR 2 HRS LATER	INSULIN TAKEN?

BLOOD SUGAR LOG

Month: ____________________ **WEEK OF:** ____________________

DATE	TIME	PRE-MEAL BLOOD SUGAR	INSULIN TAKEN?	BLOOD SUGAR 2 HRS LATER	INSULIN TAKEN?

BLOOD SUGAR LOG

Month: ______________________ **WEEK OF:** ______________________

DATE	TIME	PRE-MEAL BLOOD SUGAR	INSULIN TAKEN?	BLOOD SUGAR 2 HRS LATER	INSULIN TAKEN?

BLOOD SUGAR LOG

Month: ______________________ **WEEK OF:** ______________________

DATE	TIME	PRE-MEAL BLOOD SUGAR	INSULIN TAKEN?	BLOOD SUGAR 2 HRS LATER	INSULIN TAKEN?

BLOOD SUGAR LOG

Month: ____________________ **WEEK OF:** ____________________

DATE	TIME	PRE-MEAL BLOOD SUGAR	INSULIN TAKEN?	BLOOD SUGAR 2 HRS LATER	INSULIN TAKEN?

BLOOD SUGAR LOG

Month: ____________________ **WEEK OF:** ____________________

DATE	TIME	PRE-MEAL BLOOD SUGAR	INSULIN TAKEN?	BLOOD SUGAR 2 HRS LATER	INSULIN TAKEN?

BLOOD SUGAR LOG

Month: ____________________ **WEEK OF:** ____________________

DATE	TIME	PRE-MEAL BLOOD SUGAR	INSULIN TAKEN?	BLOOD SUGAR 2 HRS LATER	INSULIN TAKEN?

BLOOD SUGAR LOG

Month: ______________________ **WEEK OF:** ______________________

DATE	TIME	PRE-MEAL BLOOD SUGAR	INSULIN TAKEN?	BLOOD SUGAR 2 HRS LATER	INSULIN TAKEN?

BLOOD SUGAR LOG

Month: ______________________ **WEEK OF:** ______________________

DATE	TIME	PRE-MEAL BLOOD SUGAR	INSULIN TAKEN?	BLOOD SUGAR 2 HRS LATER	INSULIN TAKEN?

BLOOD SUGAR LOG

Month: ______________________ **WEEK OF:** ______________________

DATE	TIME	PRE-MEAL BLOOD SUGAR	INSULIN TAKEN?	BLOOD SUGAR 2 HRS LATER	INSULIN TAKEN?

BLOOD SUGAR LOG

Month: ____________________ WEEK OF: ____________________

DATE	TIME	PRE-MEAL BLOOD SUGAR	INSULIN TAKEN?	BLOOD SUGAR 2 HRS LATER	INSULIN TAKEN?

BLOOD SUGAR LOG

Month: ______________________ **WEEK OF:** ______________________

DATE	TIME	PRE-MEAL BLOOD SUGAR	INSULIN TAKEN?	BLOOD SUGAR 2 HRS LATER	INSULIN TAKEN?

BLOOD SUGAR LOG

Month: ______________________ **WEEK OF:** ______________________

DATE	TIME	PRE-MEAL BLOOD SUGAR	INSULIN TAKEN?	BLOOD SUGAR 2 HRS LATER	INSULIN TAKEN?

BLOOD SUGAR LOG

Month: ______________________ **WEEK OF:** ______________________

DATE	TIME	PRE-MEAL BLOOD SUGAR	INSULIN TAKEN?	BLOOD SUGAR 2 HRS LATER	INSULIN TAKEN?

BLOOD SUGAR LOG

Month: ______________________ **WEEK OF:** ______________________

DATE	TIME	PRE-MEAL BLOOD SUGAR	INSULIN TAKEN?	BLOOD SUGAR 2 HRS LATER	INSULIN TAKEN?

BLOOD SUGAR LOG

Month: ____________________ **WEEK OF:** ____________________

DATE	TIME	PRE-MEAL BLOOD SUGAR	INSULIN TAKEN?	BLOOD SUGAR 2 HRS LATER	INSULIN TAKEN?

BLOOD SUGAR LOG

Month: ____________________ **WEEK OF:** ____________________

DATE	TIME	PRE-MEAL BLOOD SUGAR	INSULIN TAKEN?	BLOOD SUGAR 2 HRS LATER	INSULIN TAKEN?

BLOOD SUGAR LOG

Month: ____________________ **WEEK OF:** ____________________

DATE	TIME	PRE-MEAL BLOOD SUGAR	INSULIN TAKEN?	BLOOD SUGAR 2 HRS LATER	INSULIN TAKEN?

BLOOD SUGAR LOG

Month: ______________________ **WEEK OF:** ______________________

DATE	TIME	PRE-MEAL BLOOD SUGAR	INSULIN TAKEN?	BLOOD SUGAR 2 HRS LATER	INSULIN TAKEN?

BLOOD SUGAR LOG

Month: ____________________ **WEEK OF:** ____________________

DATE	TIME	PRE-MEAL BLOOD SUGAR	INSULIN TAKEN?	BLOOD SUGAR 2 HRS LATER	INSULIN TAKEN?

BLOOD SUGAR LOG

Month: ____________________ **WEEK OF:** ____________________

DATE	TIME	PRE-MEAL BLOOD SUGAR	INSULIN TAKEN?	BLOOD SUGAR 2 HRS LATER	INSULIN TAKEN?

BLOOD SUGAR LOG

Month: ____________________ **WEEK OF:** ____________________

DATE	TIME	PRE-MEAL BLOOD SUGAR	INSULIN TAKEN?	BLOOD SUGAR 2 HRS LATER	INSULIN TAKEN?

BLOOD SUGAR LOG

Month: ______________________ **WEEK OF:** ______________________

DATE	TIME	PRE-MEAL BLOOD SUGAR	INSULIN TAKEN?	BLOOD SUGAR 2 HRS LATER	INSULIN TAKEN?

BLOOD SUGAR LOG

Month: ______________________________ **WEEK OF:** ______________________

DATE	TIME	PRE-MEAL BLOOD SUGAR	INSULIN TAKEN?	BLOOD SUGAR 2 HRS LATER	INSULIN TAKEN?

BLOOD SUGAR LOG

Month: ______________________ **WEEK OF:** ______________________

DATE	TIME	PRE-MEAL BLOOD SUGAR	INSULIN TAKEN?	BLOOD SUGAR 2 HRS LATER	INSULIN TAKEN?

BLOOD SUGAR LOG

Month: ______________________ **WEEK OF:** ______________________

DATE	TIME	PRE-MEAL BLOOD SUGAR	INSULIN TAKEN?	BLOOD SUGAR 2 HRS LATER	INSULIN TAKEN?

BLOOD SUGAR LOG

Month: ____________________ **WEEK OF:** ____________________

DATE	TIME	PRE-MEAL BLOOD SUGAR	INSULIN TAKEN?	BLOOD SUGAR 2 HRS LATER	INSULIN TAKEN?

BLOOD SUGAR LOG

Month: ______________________ **WEEK OF:** ______________________

DATE	TIME	PRE-MEAL BLOOD SUGAR	INSULIN TAKEN?	BLOOD SUGAR 2 HRS LATER	INSULIN TAKEN?

BLOOD SUGAR LOG

Month: ____________________ **WEEK OF:** ____________________

DATE	TIME	PRE-MEAL BLOOD SUGAR	INSULIN TAKEN?	BLOOD SUGAR 2 HRS LATER	INSULIN TAKEN?

BLOOD SUGAR LOG

Month: ______________________ **WEEK OF:** ______________________

DATE	TIME	PRE-MEAL BLOOD SUGAR	INSULIN TAKEN?	BLOOD SUGAR 2 HRS LATER	INSULIN TAKEN?

BLOOD SUGAR LOG

Month: ____________________ **WEEK OF:** ____________________

DATE	TIME	PRE-MEAL BLOOD SUGAR	INSULIN TAKEN?	BLOOD SUGAR 2 HRS LATER	INSULIN TAKEN?

BLOOD SUGAR LOG

Month: ____________________ **WEEK OF:** ____________________

DATE	TIME	PRE-MEAL BLOOD SUGAR	INSULIN TAKEN?	BLOOD SUGAR 2 HRS LATER	INSULIN TAKEN?

BLOOD SUGAR LOG

Month: ____________________ **WEEK OF:** ____________________

DATE	TIME	PRE-MEAL BLOOD SUGAR	INSULIN TAKEN?	BLOOD SUGAR 2 HRS LATER	INSULIN TAKEN?

BLOOD SUGAR LOG

Month: ____________________ **WEEK OF:** ____________________

DATE	TIME	PRE-MEAL BLOOD SUGAR	INSULIN TAKEN?	BLOOD SUGAR 2 HRS LATER	INSULIN TAKEN?

BLOOD SUGAR LOG

Month: ______________________ **WEEK OF:** ____________________

DATE	TIME	PRE-MEAL BLOOD SUGAR	INSULIN TAKEN?	BLOOD SUGAR 2 HRS LATER	INSULIN TAKEN?

BLOOD SUGAR LOG

Month: ______________________ **WEEK OF:** ______________________

DATE	TIME	PRE-MEAL BLOOD SUGAR	INSULIN TAKEN?	BLOOD SUGAR 2 HRS LATER	INSULIN TAKEN?

BLOOD SUGAR LOG

Month: ______________________ **WEEK OF:** ______________________

DATE	TIME	PRE-MEAL BLOOD SUGAR	INSULIN TAKEN?	BLOOD SUGAR 2 HRS LATER	INSULIN TAKEN?

BLOOD SUGAR LOG

Month: ______________________ **WEEK OF:** ______________________

DATE	TIME	PRE-MEAL BLOOD SUGAR	INSULIN TAKEN?	BLOOD SUGAR 2 HRS LATER	INSULIN TAKEN?

BLOOD SUGAR LOG

Month: ______________________ **WEEK OF:** ______________________

DATE	TIME	PRE-MEAL BLOOD SUGAR	INSULIN TAKEN?	BLOOD SUGAR 2 HRS LATER	INSULIN TAKEN?

BLOOD SUGAR LOG

Month: ______________________ **WEEK OF:** ______________________

DATE	TIME	PRE-MEAL BLOOD SUGAR	INSULIN TAKEN?	BLOOD SUGAR 2 HRS LATER	INSULIN TAKEN?

BLOOD SUGAR LOG

Month: ____________________ **WEEK OF:** ____________________

DATE	TIME	PRE-MEAL BLOOD SUGAR	INSULIN TAKEN?	BLOOD SUGAR 2 HRS LATER	INSULIN TAKEN?

BLOOD SUGAR LOG

Month: ______________________ **WEEK OF:** ______________________

DATE	TIME	PRE-MEAL BLOOD SUGAR	INSULIN TAKEN?	BLOOD SUGAR 2 HRS LATER	INSULIN TAKEN?

BLOOD SUGAR LOG

Month: ______________________ **WEEK OF:** ______________________

DATE	TIME	PRE-MEAL BLOOD SUGAR	INSULIN TAKEN?	BLOOD SUGAR 2 HRS LATER	INSULIN TAKEN?

BLOOD SUGAR LOG

Month: ______________________ WEEK OF: ______________________

DATE	TIME	PRE-MEAL BLOOD SUGAR	INSULIN TAKEN?	BLOOD SUGAR 2 HRS LATER	INSULIN TAKEN?

BLOOD SUGAR LOG

Month: ______________________ **WEEK OF:** ______________________

DATE	TIME	PRE-MEAL BLOOD SUGAR	INSULIN TAKEN?	BLOOD SUGAR 2 HRS LATER	INSULIN TAKEN?

BLOOD SUGAR LOG

Month: ____________________ **WEEK OF:** ____________________

DATE	TIME	PRE-MEAL BLOOD SUGAR	INSULIN TAKEN?	BLOOD SUGAR 2 HRS LATER	INSULIN TAKEN?

BLOOD SUGAR LOG

Month: ______________________ WEEK OF: ______________________

DATE	TIME	PRE-MEAL BLOOD SUGAR	INSULIN TAKEN?	BLOOD SUGAR 2 HRS LATER	INSULIN TAKEN?

BLOOD SUGAR LOG

Month: ______________________ **WEEK OF:** ______________________

DATE	TIME	PRE-MEAL BLOOD SUGAR	INSULIN TAKEN?	BLOOD SUGAR 2 HRS LATER	INSULIN TAKEN?

BLOOD SUGAR LOG

Month: ______________________ **WEEK OF:** ______________________

DATE	TIME	PRE-MEAL BLOOD SUGAR	INSULIN TAKEN?	BLOOD SUGAR 2 HRS LATER	INSULIN TAKEN?

BLOOD SUGAR LOG

Month: ______________________ **WEEK OF:** ______________________

DATE	TIME	PRE-MEAL BLOOD SUGAR	INSULIN TAKEN?	BLOOD SUGAR 2 HRS LATER	INSULIN TAKEN?

BLOOD SUGAR LOG

Month: ____________________ **WEEK OF:** ____________________

DATE	TIME	PRE-MEAL BLOOD SUGAR	INSULIN TAKEN?	BLOOD SUGAR 2 HRS LATER	INSULIN TAKEN?

BLOOD SUGAR LOG

Month: ______________________ **WEEK OF:** ______________________

DATE	TIME	PRE-MEAL BLOOD SUGAR	INSULIN TAKEN?	BLOOD SUGAR 2 HRS LATER	INSULIN TAKEN?

BLOOD SUGAR LOG

Month: ______________________ **WEEK OF:** ______________________

DATE	TIME	PRE-MEAL BLOOD SUGAR	INSULIN TAKEN?	BLOOD SUGAR 2 HRS LATER	INSULIN TAKEN?

BLOOD SUGAR LOG

Month: ______________________ **WEEK OF:** ______________________

DATE	TIME	PRE-MEAL BLOOD SUGAR	INSULIN TAKEN?	BLOOD SUGAR 2 HRS LATER	INSULIN TAKEN?

BLOOD SUGAR LOG

Month: ______________________ **WEEK OF:** ______________________

DATE	TIME	PRE-MEAL BLOOD SUGAR	INSULIN TAKEN?	BLOOD SUGAR 2 HRS LATER	INSULIN TAKEN?

BLOOD SUGAR LOG

Month: ______________________ **WEEK OF:** ______________________

DATE	TIME	PRE-MEAL BLOOD SUGAR	INSULIN TAKEN?	BLOOD SUGAR 2 HRS LATER	INSULIN TAKEN?

BLOOD SUGAR LOG

Month: ______________________ **WEEK OF:** ______________________

DATE	TIME	PRE-MEAL BLOOD SUGAR	INSULIN TAKEN?	BLOOD SUGAR 2 HRS LATER	INSULIN TAKEN?

BLOOD SUGAR LOG

Month: ______________________ **WEEK OF:** ______________________

DATE	TIME	PRE-MEAL BLOOD SUGAR	INSULIN TAKEN?	BLOOD SUGAR 2 HRS LATER	INSULIN TAKEN?

BLOOD SUGAR LOG

Month: ______________________________ **WEEK OF:** ______________________

DATE	TIME	PRE-MEAL BLOOD SUGAR	INSULIN TAKEN?	BLOOD SUGAR 2 HRS LATER	INSULIN TAKEN?

BLOOD SUGAR LOG

Month: ______________________ **WEEK OF:** ______________________

DATE	TIME	PRE-MEAL BLOOD SUGAR	INSULIN TAKEN?	BLOOD SUGAR 2 HRS LATER	INSULIN TAKEN?

BLOOD SUGAR LOG

Month: ______________________________ **WEEK OF:** ______________________

DATE	TIME	PRE-MEAL BLOOD SUGAR	INSULIN TAKEN?	BLOOD SUGAR 2 HRS LATER	INSULIN TAKEN?

NOTES

Name:

NOTES

Name:

STAY ORGANIZED
STAY EMPOWERED

Want a FREE Diabetic Meal Planner?

Get your free printable, plus health tips to help you stay on track.

Visit: www.mealplan.adalynnjames.com

Enter your name & email to download instantly!

Enjoying this logbook?

Your honest review helps others find this book and supports businesses like ours.

Please take a minute to leave a review on Amazon. We read every single one! Scan the QR code below.

https://bit.ly/BloodSugarLogBookReview

— DigiMedical, by Adalynn James Publishing

Digi Medical

ADALYNN JAMES

Made in the USA
Monee, IL
04 November 2026

67379623R00066